About me

My name is Franciol Pikert and I have a strong passion for helping individuals get their life back on the healthy track.

Acknowledgments

I would like to thank my personal trainer and my dietician, Roger Suik.

About this book

In this book, I talk about the 4 most important things you can do to improve your diet for weight loss.

Content page

Avoid Carbohydrates

While we can get by without sugar, it would be very hard to take out starches completely from your eating regimen. Sugars are the body's principle wellspring of vitality. In their nonattendance, your body will utilize protein and fat for vitality.

It might likewise be difficult to get enough fiber, which is essential for a sound stomach related framework and to counteract clogging.

Solid wellsprings of sugars, for example, bland sustenances, vegetables, organic products, vegetables and lower fat dairy items are likewise a vital wellspring of supplements, for example, calcium, iron and B vitamins.

Removing sugars from your eating routine could put you at

expanded danger of an insufficiency in specific supplements, prompting medical issues, except if you're ready to compensate for the dietary deficit with solid substitutes.

Supplanting sugars with fats and higher fat wellsprings of protein could expand your admission of soaked fat, which can raise the measure of cholesterol in your blood – a hazard factor for coronary illness.

When you are low on glucose, the body separates put away fat to change over it into vitality. This procedure causes a development of ketones in the blood, bringing about ketosis.

Ketosis because of a low sugar eating regimen can be connected, in any event for the time being, to cerebral pains, shortcoming, queasiness, lack of hydration, unsteadiness, and fractiousness.

Attempt to confine the measure of sugary sustenances you eat and rather incorporate more advantageous wellsprings of starch in your eating regimen, for example, whole grains, potatoes, vegetables, organic products, vegetables and lower fat dairy items.

Read the British Dietetic Association's survey of low-carb diets, including the paleo,

Dukan, Atkins, and South Beach

abstains from food.

Load Up On Saturated Fats

For quite a while, we were on the whole to avoid fats, and general stores reacted with an endless supply of items with the "without fat" mark embellished on it.

Be that as it may, you will commit a gigantic error by keeping away from this supplement on the off chance that you are endeavoring to keep up your weight.

First of all, fats assume a critical part in our body, going about as a vitality hold, ensuring our organs and helping the body ingest and process supplements. That is the reason we require a few fats in our eating regimen.

As indicated by the Health Promotion Board, fats should make up 25 for every penny to 30 for each penny of our aggregate vitality admission.

On the off chance that you are attempting to shed the pounds, the fat that you expend should originate from unsaturated sources, (for example, monounsaturated fat).

Cases of such nourishments incorporate fish, seeds, nuts and olive oil.

Other than enhancing heart wellbeing by evacuating low-thickness lipoprotein cholesterol - the "terrible" cholesterol - from the veins, these solid nourishments additionally enable you to consume fat without cutting calories.

The body requires three macronutrients for vitality - starches, proteins, and fats.

A gram of fat gives the body double the measure of the vitality of the other two.

Once the vitality got from sugars is spent, the body would divert to the calories from fats as a wellspring of vitality, inclining out the body.

Analysts at the Washington University School of Medicine in St. Louis, Missouri, found that obstinate "old" fat put away in the body's fringe tissues around the midsection, thighs and rear end can't be scorched without

the utilization of "new" dietary
fats.

Whenever devoured, the
supplement separates the
current fat by actuating PPAR-
alpha (the protein that revs up
digestion) and fat-consuming
the liver.

Drink Plenty
Of Water

A large portion of the examinations recorded beneath took a gander at the impact of drinking one, 0.5 liter (17 oz) serving of water. Drinking water expands the measure of calories you consume, which is known as resting vitality use.

In grown-ups, resting vitality consumption has been appeared to increment by 24–30% inside 10 minutes of drinking water. This keeps going no less than an hour.

Supporting this, one investigation of overweight and stout kids found a 25% expansion in resting vitality use subsequent to drinking cool water. An investigation of overweight ladies inspected the impacts of expanding water admission to more than 1 liter (34 oz) every day. They found that over a year time span, this brought about an additional 2 kg (4.4 lbs) of weight reduction.

Since these ladies didn't roll out any way of life improvements but to drink more water, these outcomes are exceptionally amazing.

Also, both of these investigations demonstrate that drinking 0.5

liters (17 oz) of water brings about an additional 23 calories consumed. On a yearly premise, that aggregates up to about 17,000 calories — or more than 2 kg (4.4 lbs) of fat.

A few different investigations have checked overweight individuals who drank 1-1.5 liters (34– 50 oz) of water day by day for half a month. They found a noteworthy lessening in weight, weight file (BMI), midsection periphery and muscle versus fat.

These outcomes might be much greater when the water is chilly. When you drink cool water, your body utilizes additional calories to warm the water up to body temperature.

A few people assert that drinking water before a supper diminishes hunger.

There really is by all accounts some fact behind this, however only in moderately aged and more established grown-ups. Investigations of more established grown-ups have demonstrated that drinking water before every dinner may build weight reduction by 2 kg (4.4 lbs) over a 12-week time frame.

In one investigation, moderately aged overweight and fat members who drank water before every feast lost 44% more weight, contrasted with a gathering that did not drink more water.

Another investigation additionally demonstrated that drinking water before breakfast decreased the measure of calories expended amid the dinner by 13%.

In spite of the fact that this might be extremely gainful for moderately aged and more seasoned individuals, investigations of more youthful people have not demonstrated the same great decrease in calorie consumption.

Eat Vegetables

Get in shape? Live more? Possibly your mother was correct when she instructed you to eat your vegetables. Luckily, vegetables are a critical part of the Atkins Nutritional Approach.

Indeed, even in Induction, 12 to 15 grams day by day of Net Carbs should originate from up to six measures of a plate of mixed greens and up to two measures of cooked vegetables (contingent upon which vegetables you pick).

Your decisions turn out to be considerably more ample as you travel through resulting periods of Atkins. Read on for more reasons why you have to eat your vegetables.

Vegetables help keep you full for more. The fiber and water in vegetables top you off much more productively than eating prepared carbs that are inadequate in fiber.

Consolidating vegetables with protein and solid fats will keep you fulfilled until it's the ideal opportunity for your next supper.

Vegetables help avert plunges and spikes in your vitality levels. By and by, the fiber in vegetables controls your glucose.

In case you're eating all your allocated vegetables every day, you shouldn't encounter that late-evening vitality droop (and yearnings for sugar) that you may experience when eating handled starches.

Vegetables enable you to live more. Various investigations demonstrate that an eating regimen wealthy in an assortment of vegetables may help diminish the solidifying of supply routes, help bring down cholesterol levels and help avoid irritation, a segment of numerous degenerative sicknesses including heftiness, diabetes, coronary illness and Alzheimer's.

Scientists trust the cell reinforcements (vitamins C and E, in addition to selenium and the carotenoids) might be mostly in charge of this impact.

Vegetables are a definitive sustenance substitution. You

can't turn out badly when you supplant shoddy nourishment and handled sugars, which are regularly brimming with unfortunate fats and lacking in supplements, with supplement thick sustenances like vegetables, which contain fiber, cancer prevention agents, and vitamins.

Vegetables enable you to get in shape. Vegetables have a tendency to bring down in calories, yet pack a way more great punch with regards to keeping you sound and full for more.

This all methods you may have a tendency to eat fewer calories, while as yet feeling fulfilled, if not more fulfilled, than when you depend on bundled nourishments and sustenances without supplements.

www.ingramcontent.com/pod-product-compliance
Lightning Source LLC
Chambersburg PA
CBHW070100260726
48658CB00002B/922